Natural Hair Care
Step-by-Step Guide To Healthy Curly Natural Hair

Meloney Washington

Good Hair Coaching, LLC

Clearwater, FL

Meloney Washington/Good Hair Coaching
100 Belcher Road Unit 8428
Clearwater, Florida 33758
(888) 383-0985

www.goodhaircoaching.com

Special thanks to my book coach Stefanie Newell and editor Sarah Strowbridge of http://howtowriteabookthatsells.com and editor Karen Rodgers of http://critiqueyourbook.com

Natural Hair Care/Meloney Washington. -- 1st ed.

I dedicate this book to my Mom and Dad

Although I wasn't raised with my mom and dad, I do appreciate the life they chose for me. My parents couldn't give me a lot, but they gave me my good genes to wear with pride. I have an open mind to think and make choices that affect me positively. I have an open heart that genuinely loves and cares about people and for the bad days, I have inherited their sense of humor to inject the best form of natural medicine "laughter" into others and myself. I have never complained about what my parents couldn't give me. They both deserve my honor and my respect for simply choosing to give me a LIFE. A life that has offered me the opportunity to be the best person that I can be. I love them even more for that.

Mel

CONTENTS

LETTER FROM A FRIEND

Meloney,

My friend you have inspired me in your pursuit of healthy, attractive natural hair.

We have known one another for many years, and have gone through the trends together and there have been many to say the least.

I have admired your transition from chemically treated to natural, all the while managing to maintain a coiffed and polished look! You have managed to do so while raising two wonderful children, nurturing a wonderful marriage and giving of your time to our friendship and countless others; you have proven that it can be done with diligence and patience.

Readers,

As you read this manual on how to go natural and maintain a beautiful stylish look, it may seem a difficult task and in some cases it is. The in-between stage from chemical to natural is a difficult stage, but you can get through it if you stay focused on your goal. I am confident you can make it through to the beautiful end! As you navigate your way through and look at the pictures, it may seem daunting and tough, but know that you too can accomplish this with a determined mindset and your hands and heart ready and willing to do the work.

Naomi Tillman

FOREWORD

My name is Angela "Overkill" Hill. I'm a professional MMA and Muay Thai fighter, Muay Thai World Champion, first Black woman to be signed to the UFC and current champion in Invicta FC. I've managed to build quite a following. Not just from my relentless fighting style, but my unique look and cool fro-hawk as well. In the last 3 years, I've done a lifetime's worth of getting dolled up and having my hair pulled, blown out and straightened for promotional events and photoshoots. Trying to look glamourous is almost as tiring as fighting itself. When Meloney Washington contacted me to write the foreword of her book, I was honored. I guess I've been doing something right!

When someone mentions the term "going natural," I get this feeling of nostalgia because there aren't many women of African descent in my career. Occasionally I get messages from fans about hair care and, honestly, I've just been winging it for years. Reading Meloney Washington's book not only legitimized in my head some of the techniques I've been using, but it taught me some useful tips for every day styles and tips for when I want to look like a movie star.

I've struggled with hair care since I decided to stop perming my hair as a teenager. I was an artsy high schooler, listening to the likes of Erykah Badu, India Arie and Lauryn Hill (no relation, though I'd always pretend that she was my big sis on the radio), and I was totally inspired to embrace my natural self. That and the fact that my hair was looking thinner with every perm! I knew I had to make a change or risk ending up rocking a Crypt Keeper-esque hairstyle from continuing to use harsh straightening chemicals.

After two strand twisting my hair for about a year, I made the big chop as a freshman in college. I was always the girl with the long hair, so it was a huge deal for me. I still recall my family members saying, "Why did you cut off all that beautiful hair?!" I felt more free, but at the same time every hairstyle was an experiment. Some were successful and some went terribly wrong. I was lucky enough to be in a forgiving environment like art school. There, you could show up with leaves in your hair and no one would bat an eye. My mother on the other hand was working in an office in DC for over 15 years when she decided to loc her hair, and was subsequently fired for her appearance. She was smart enough to sue and was back on her feet in no time, but I'm sure many people have crazy stories of how they were suddenly treated differently whilst trying to figure out their new natural hair.

We live in a different time now where the natural look has become way more accepted and, even though I've had my hair natural for over a decade, reading through Meloney Washington's book gave me all sorts of tips and tricks I hadn't tried yet. It's like a recipe book for the curly, kinky and tangle headed woman. I really enjoyed the "How To" sections dealing with shampooing, conditioning and straightening, because these are the tasks where I cause the most damage and break-age to my hair. Also, now that my job is basically working out 6 days a week and sparring and grappling with opponents, I am constantly having to wash the grossness out of my hair and dryness is a huge issue for me. I really found the dry hair syndrome (DHS) sections helpful and will be going back to them to try different recipes until I find out what works for me.

This book is an easy read and Meloney Washington does a great job of telling you what ingredients to look for without sounding like a commercial for certain products. She also shares her own experiences, which is always helpful for the newly natural. I can't wait to try out all the methods I've over-looked before now and hope that this book is able to inspire others to experiment and feel beautiful with their hair. I wish her all the best with this book!

www.sherdog.com/fighter/Angela-Hill

STYLES, PRODUCTS AND GROWTH REGIMENS

Are you unable to achieve the attractive look you desire with your natural hair? Are you tired of struggling to transition your hair with no success? Are you clueless about how to style and maintain your own healthy hair? Are you stuck wearing wigs and weaves because you don't know what else to do with your hair?

Whether you are new to the natural hair game or are already in it, if you are having a hard time handling your children's hair or keeping your own hair healthy and growing, *Natural Hair Care: Step-by-Step Guide to Healthy Curly Natural Hair* is the playbook for real success.

While reading this book you will discover:

- How to maintain your own hair
- Ways to avoid the pitfalls of trial and error
- Basic "get up and go" protective styles just right for you
- How to maintain healthy hair with basic transition styles
- How to feel attractive at every stage during the process
- Tame your hair and your child's hair with proven regimens
- Learn protective style techniques to sleep, work out, swim and have healthy hair

You will learn how to take care of your hair properly, so you end up with your own gorgeous hair! After you finish this book, you will know how to maintain healthy hair with basic regimens and master basic techniques for an everyday, professional salon look.

In each chapter you will get information and instructions that allow you to learn essential regimens that include properly washing, co-washing, conditioning and moisturizing. You will also read about techniques for proper style takedowns, heatless sets, stretching and more.

Before we get started, let me share my own hair story so you can better understand why this book was necessary.

My Hair Story

I didn't choose this natural hair path as a business; it kind of found its way to me. Back in 1998, while working as a financial service agent, I was blessed to meet Joyce C. Mitchell, previous owner of Anako-Nappy Beauty Salon in St. Petersburg, Florida. This salon specialized in the care and upkeep of Sista Locs. Joyce had a passion for natural hair, and the encouragement she gave for cultural awareness opened the door for me to embrace my natural beauty. Joyce left us in 2006, and although I never knew her personally outside of this industry, I will forever be grateful to her for introducing me to my *HAIRstorical* roots.

In my pursuit of nappiness, one of the first things I discovered is that the truth about having naturally good hair is, literally, NO LYE! I was already braiding my hair and working part time braiding and wrapping for others. When my daughter and I decided that we would go natural and convert to wearing the sister locs, we discovered something truly amazing—our BEAUTIFUL NATURAL HAIR TEXTURE! Once it had all grown in, we fell in love with it and decided to keep it just the way it was.

After a while, my daughter and I wanted to be able to wear our curls out and have more style options. We took some really bad advice and went to a professional salon. We had them put a texturizer in our hair, thinking that it would allow our hair to be more manageable for styling. Boy, were we wrong! To make that long story short, a couple of months later my hair became damaged to the point that I was losing my beautiful long locs in patches. There was nothing left for me to do but cut it off and start all over again.

Fast forward a year later and my locs were coming back longer and stronger. I couldn't believe how quickly the time went by. I branched out and started to assist more women in wearing natural styles and transitioning. I found that there were lots of others out there who were attempting to transition without good results. Women were giving up early in the game due to their frustration. While assisting these women in their transitioning, and seeing some great success from the one-on-one coaching I was offering, I wanted to help even more.

Now armed with the experience of having transitioned twice, once via growing out my relaxer and the second time around having to do a big chop, I began to research ways to develop my hair maintenance skills. I studied natural hair and became a self-proclaimed professional "knottiologist." As a Licensed Natural Hair Specialist, I decided to provide hands-on training and motivation in an educational setting for would-be natural hair stylists so that more women could have good hair success.

Initially it was very difficult to transition and then maintain my own natural hair. But through trial and error I learned to properly care for my hair, and eventually experienced healthy hair growth. Oh, how I wish I had known what I know now back when I was transitioning the first time. It was with that thought that the idea of Good Hair Coaching was born.

I started Good Hair Coaching LLC for all the naturals out there. Because like a lot of you, I had to struggle to transition and once I transitioned completely, then came the issues with the upkeep for my own natural hair.

I also jumped on the bandwagon with everyone else who was trying every product out there, which only led me to wearing weaves and wigs because I had no idea what else to do. Finally, I even went to licensed cosmetologists, who were proficient in their work, but did not specialize in the care and maintenance of my natural curls.

After having to transition twice, I decided to take those hard lessons that I learned from my experiences and create the ultimate "how to" coaching guide that I wish had been available back when I needed it.

Having a book like this could have directed me how to do the things I needed to do to make my hair manageable, and could have saved me a lot of time and undue stress.

In the "How To" sections on regimens and techniques in *Natural Hair Care: Step-by-Step Guide to Healthy Curly Natural Hair* you will find page after page of easy to follow steps designed to show you how to do to your own hair. You will also find simple answers to simple questions, as well as tips, facts, quotes and more from leading natural hair care industry professional knottiologists, stylists, bloggers, vloggers and authors.

What sets Good Hair Coaching apart in this industry is that the programs offered are not overly focused on product pushing. They are designed to teach students to choose proper products, learn regimens and master techniques for their own personal good hair upkeep.

Although I have become a natural hair advocate, this good hair coach is not at all a "Napturalista Nazi." As a former relaxed woman, in addition to training those who want to transition, I am also qualified to offer very helpful information for my "Relaxed Sistas," and those who desire to use natural hair care products, services and protective hairstyle maintenance techniques to maintain and grow healthy hair.

Now, you won't learn any ancient hidden secrets for natural hair care, but you will discover some good ol' fashioned, long forgotten, back to basics techniques, skills, recipes and grandma's tricks and tips with a new school twist.

Finally! You can look in the mirror every day and love what you see. A naturally strong, bold, empowered, flawless woman who is ready to conquer the world! So grab this book while you still can, dive right in and come out turning heads everywhere you go with your beautiful natural hair!

CHAPTER ONE

ABOUT NATURAL HAIR CARE

What you should know about natural hair care

There is no right or wrong choice for your good hair. The benefits come from knowing how to have healthy hair no matter which way you decide to go.

Contrary to popular opinion, our natural textured hair is not as difficult as we make it out to be in our minds. Even though natural is not for everyone, it is more beneficial for some than others. However, being natural involves a mindset transition as well as making a personal choice. Most of us never knew our natural hair because we were not raised to wear it—we were never taught how to care for it. Therefore, it is foreign to us. To see it as "good" is out of reach in our own minds. Transforming what is "good" in your mind is critical. As your hair is changing, your way of thinking must change with it, or you absolutely will not stay the course.

First: Consider the cost for maintenance and management of natural and straight hair.

Second: Choose the best solution, natural or straight.

Third: Make a decision to start the journey to your good hair.

Cost, Maintenance and Management of Natural and Straight Hair

How much does it cost to maintain natural vs. straight hair?

That is determined by what is right for your type and texture. All the commercialism surrounding hair care in general has led us all to become product junkies that need to try everything on the market to find success. Your natural locks were never expensive to care for from the beginning, but the benefit of being natural is that prices can range from high end designer care to "low-key-low-cost" care. It all boils down to finding what truly works for your tresses in the price range that is comfortable for you.

Is it difficult to manage natural or straight hair?

Your hair requires some maintenance either way. If you can master the basics of good hair care—proper washing, conditioning, detangling, trimming and styling—you win! Using the right techniques and regular regimens will assure healthy strong hair. Research is half the battle, and that is why I've created this step-by-step coaching guide. You won't lose time and money trying to figure it all out on your own.

It can be difficult to manage your hair. If you have no idea what you are doing, the process will be challenging and more difficult than it should be. Do you fear not having an attractive or professional look, or do you believe that your hair is so bad that it can never be good? There could be several reasons for the issues that we have. However in many cases, products that are not compatible for your type and texture can cause the hair to lose its natural health and hydration.

We have been taught from youth to believe that under the texturizers and relaxers is hard to handle, bad nappy hair. I don't know what nappy hair is, but what I do know is that our strands naturally will curl and coil as it grows until it intertwines back into itself or other stands. For the most part, when we handle those curls or coils from the root incorrectly, we tend to pull down, create tension and cause them to become knots. I like to believe that contrary to popular opinion, my hair does not get nappy, it gets knotty. It is possible to undo knots, train them and develop your strands to do what they should do naturally, which is to coil, curl or wave.

One of the biggest challenges to transitioning back to natural is that every woman wants to look her best during the transition and beyond. Because some of us have been relaxed even before we had ever seen or got to know the type and texture of our hair, we have no idea how to get the look we desire, so we give up.

What is the best way to get back to your natural hair texture?

There are two ways to go natural. There is the transitioning method and the big chop. The transitioning method allows you to gradually grow your hair out, which means that you will keep your relaxed texture while you grow the natural roots in via transition. You could also cut the relaxed hair off right away, which is referred to as, "the big chop." There is no best way, just the right way for you.

By using styles that do not require daily grooming and regular use of heat, you can keep the hair from having a lot of damage during the process.

Depending upon the type and texture of your hair, complete transitions can take from 6 months to a year or more, provided you are not doing the big chop.

Do I grow out my perm or chemically treated hair?

Keep in mind that half way through the transition is where most give up. Working with two different textures on your head will cause many emotions, so beware! Just remember that you cannot treat natural hair like it is processed. If you choose this method, then the best way to do it and not have a significant amount of damage during the process would be to:

1. Use good transition and protective styles.
2. Keep your hair trimmed as it grows to keep the hair from breaking and splitting on the ends.
3. Choose two or three go-to styles that will keep you from constantly manipulating your hair and keep you from getting bored, especially if you occasionally like being able to change up your look.

You will find more information about transitioning maintenance, protective styles and "go to" styles in Chapter 5.

Should I do the big chop?

If you want to become an instant natural, it is as easy as chopping it all off down to the new growth and just getting started. Committing to regular regimens and techniques is going to be the key to real success and healthy hair growth. Pay attention to the regimens and techniques found in Chapters 4 and 5 to fit you and your lifestyle.

Doing the big chop can be scary for some, especially if you are comfortable with seeing yourself with medium to long hair. Then there are the hecklers who will always have something to say, but nothing at all productive to contribute. Can you stand it? That is the question. You will need to be strong to get through that rough patch. The most important thing that you can do for yourself is - be confident about your look, and make sure that everyone around you knows you love it!

Remain processed or be straight?

Straight talk! All the back and forth about which hair is the best is absolutely ridiculous. People transition for many reasons. One reason being that they have had a bad experience with being able to maintain strong, healthy processed hair. For others, it's just a personal decision. The beauty of ethnic hair is that we can choose either and still have the benefit of wearing either straight or curly. Flat ironing and hot pressing have come a long way, and we can go straight whenever we want!

The issue among most processed women is not that different from those who are natural. We all desire to have healthy hair that grows. Like the naturals, learning how to properly care for processed hair is essential. Some have gone from stylist to stylist trying to find someone who could really make it happen.

I could have decided to keep my processed hair because, to be honest with you, I had no real issues with it. I maintained healthy strong hair at a decent length. Although I would have liked to have my hair longer, it was not a pressing issue for me because I was happy with my hair being healthy at the time.

Believe me, I had my days of salon hopping. But by mastering the upkeep myself, I came to realize I could better educate my stylist on my hair needs. Think about it, the only way that a doctor can help you with whatever is bothering you is by first getting to know you through the questionnaire that you fill out in his office waiting room. Why is this information important? Because nobody knows your body better than you, so why not know and understand your hair the same way? With that knowledge, it doesn't matter if you or a stylist does your hair, you will always have amazing results.

My point is that all hair is good hair and has the ability to grow and be healthy. Transitioning to natural was an educated, personal decision that was right for me. I do believe that natural NO LYE is good hair, but for those who still can't choose natural, relax! It's still good hair. The regimens and techniques found in this book will benefit both my natural and relaxed sistas.

Make a decision

Now, what are you going to do?

Prior to making your decision, you need to know that contrary to popular opinion, all textures of hair will grow and all textures of hair require some time and work. For good results you need to be willing to learn and understand your own hair.

Whether you're going to move forward with transitioning, continue being natural or remain in your relaxed tresses, the information found here was put together to assist you no matter what you decide. The solution is to choose what is best for you.

Bottom line is, to make a decision and start your journey to good hair!

Get to know your own hair

One of the first things you should do is take the time to get to know your hair. You will learn a lot from other people with similar hair textures, but keep in mind that what's good for them is not always going to be what is good for you. Learn about your own hair!

I'm going to be honest with you; I personally do not get into the hair typing of today. 1a, 4d, 3d TV or whatever else there is. I believe in the old school hair typing, which is shape, texture and feel of the hair. I get confused with all the extras, so I want to make it easy for you too.

Shape and Texture

- The three general shapes are curly, wavy and straight
- The three texture types are fine, medium and thick

Symptoms of Dry Hair

- Hard and brittle to touch
- Tiny flakes or dry skin from your scalp
- Hair sheds and breaks

Symptoms of Oily Hair

- Strands feel slick or greasy
- Heavy flaking from the scalp
- Pimples on the forehead close to the hairline

Symptoms of Normal Hair

- No flaking from the scalp
- No excessive oiliness
- No excessive dryness

Personal Hair Evaluation

Let's do an evaluation of your hair. Start by answering the following questions:

- How does it feel?
- What does it look like?
- Is it short, medium or long in length?
- What happens when you pull it away from your scalp and let it go?
- Does it fall straight down, recoil or spring back to the scalp or something in between?
- Would you describe the shape of your hair strand as straight, curly or wavy?

Personal Hair Testing

Now do a test of your hair's porosity to determine its ability to absorb water and other chemicals in the shaft of the hair. Hair with high porosity can absorb a lot of water, but will also release moisture very quickly. Low porosity hair will hold on to moisture longer, but the hair will not easily pull in water. Follow the simple steps below:

1. Fill a glass or bowl with room temperature water.
2. Take a couple of strands of your clean hair and put them in the water.
3. Watch it for 2-4 minutes. If your hair sinks immediately, it has high porosity.

Coach's Tip: It is best to evaluate your hair while it is dry and then again when it is wet. For accurate results, use clean hair when conducting the porosity testing.

NOTES:

_____

_____

_____

_____

_____

_____

_____

_____

CHAPTER TWO

PRODUCTS AND NATURAL REMEDIES

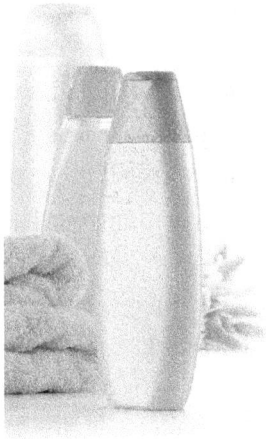

What to look for in your products?

"You know, I don't know," said Madea. Science and chemistry were not my best topics, so some serious thought went into how to share this information with you. I won't spend a lot of time on this because there are so many vloggers, bloggers and authors before me that have provided this information in much greater detail. In fact, Audrey Davis-Sivasothy is one resource that will give you the mother load of information about textured hair in her book, *The Science of Black Hair*. So I don't end up beating a dead horse with the same information, I have a KISS for you. I will **Keep It Super Simple.**

Hair thrives when it is clean, conditioned and moisturized. The commercialism around hair products, in my opinion, is overkill. It is interesting to note that for many years, most hair care companies didn't even consider ethnic hair when marketing their products. Now they have somehow become experts and have managed to create dedicated lines of product just for ethnic hair. Now, I'm not hating on the players, I'm just not feeling the game.

What you should remember is that just because it says it's for ethnic hair does not mean that it is the best. If you have something that is working for you, then you should keep it in your regimen. Always stay within your budget, stick to those products that work for you and not everything advertised or shown in YouTube videos. More important than that, pay attention to how you apply product to your hair. It's been said that when using products, less is more. Personally, I am still working on that one. I'm a bit heavy handed and still have to work on how much product I put into my own hair. So don't do me, just do you.

Most of us get on the product rampage because we can't seem to find something to keep our hair from being so dry. Is your natural hair so dry that when you try to comb it, it sounds like you're biting an apple? You should be bent over laughing now. Ok, I am no comedian, but I thought that was funny. We all have had Dry Hair Syndrome (DHS) at some point.

Well, I have good news and I have bad news. The bad news first, so that the good news can make you feel better. Bad news is, there is no one amazing product that can help you with that. Now, the good news is that there is a way to make it all better right now. That's right, it does not take some time-consuming process to give your hair what it needs to hold moisture. You're going to learn just how simple it is to "loc in moisture" right here in this book! I will explain more in detail in chapter 4.

To shampoo or not to shampoo, that is the question. I will say that is totally up to you. Shampoo generally leaves curly hair frizzy and out of control. If you've been doing research, then you already know that ammonium laureth sulfate, ammonium lauryl sulfate, sodium laureth sulfate, sodium lauryl sulfate blah blah blah (whew), are all drying sulfates that will damage the hair. All you really need to know is, if you are going to use shampoo, make sure that the cleansers are mild. According to the *Curly Girl Guide* book by Lorraine Massey, mild cleansers (i.e. cocamidopropyl betaine or coco betaine) can be used occasionally without causing any harm to the hair.

I personally do not shampoo my hair except on occasions when there is heavy product build up, beach salt water or chlorine from the pool. I was using the "no poo" method long before I ever heard about it. The "no poo" method, aka co-wash, is simply the process of cleansing your hair with a leave-in conditioner. A lot of natural experts recommend doing this versus shampoo. I must agree that co-washing is very gentle on the hair. A lot of naturals and relaxed clients have seen healthy hair using this process.

When it comes to moisture, I am the biggest fan of it for the hair. In doing research about moisture, I found some very interesting information from Fran of Heyfranhey.com. She wrote an amazing article, *"Winter Hair Care: Moisturizing Oils vs Sealing Oils,"* that explained the difference between the two types of oils. The aforementioned article was easy to understand and just made sense. It explained that only 3 oils—coconut oil, olive oil and avocado oil—have a molecular structure small enough to actually penetrate the hair shaft and induce moisture. Other oils like Jamaican castor oil, grape seed oil, and jojoba oil will sit on top of the strand, coating the cuticle, and sealing in moisture. An understanding of both types will ensure an effective hair regimen. But, as always, no two heads are alike. It is helpful to try different oils and methods to see which works best for your particular hair type.

If you feel oil isn't sufficient to hold in or seal in enough moisture, try a soft but thick butter, like raw shea butter. If you feel butters and oils aren't for you, try sealing your hair after applying your leave-in with Pure Aloe Vera Juice. Its acidity is perfect for closing the cuticle. Please check out that article, *"Winter Hair Care: Moisturizing Oils vs Sealing Oils"* if you are interested in learning more.

Shampoos, Conditioners and Moisturizers

Choose the proper shampoo and conditioner based on pH factors

Potential Hydrogen (pH) describes the acidic and alkaline volume ratio in your shampoo, and is measured on a scale from 1 to 14. The lower the pH reading, the more acidic and oxygen deprived the fluid is. The higher the pH reading, the more alkaline and oxygen rich the fluid is.

A pH-balanced shampoo usually describes a shampoo that is chemically balanced to clean your hair without stripping it of natural moisture and oil. It rates between 5 and 7 on the pH scale. 6.5 to 7 is a normal range for pH-balanced shampoos.

A pH scale 1 to 3 or 11 to 14 can potentially damage the skin and hair.

pH Scale 1 to 5 – Acidic Products

This scale includes the following products:

- Lemon rinses
- Color rinses
- Hydrogen peroxide (used in permanent coloring)
- Neutralizers (for chemical straighteners)

pH Scale 5 to 9 – Alkaline Products

This scale includes the following products:

- Soap shampoos (olive or coconut oil based)
- Conditioners
- Cream rinses
- Anti-dandruff shampoos
- Hair preparations: pomades, hair grease, petroleum, or beeswax-based products

- Semi-permanent color
- Permanent color

pH Scale 10 to 14

This scale includes the following products:

- Chemical straighteners
- Bleaches (super destructive products)

Most manufactured shampoos are pH balanced

High alkaline clarifying shampoos are not pH balanced. They are designed to remove buildup from hard water, gels, sprays, mousses, pool chemicals etc. They also have a lot of perfumes and other additives. You don't need these unless you have the above conditions.

Shampoos are used to cleanse the scalp of dust, dirt, grease and oil.

Things to know if you're going to use a shampoo regimen:

- Generally leaves curly hair frizzy
- Generally leaves straight hair dry
- Mild shampoo cleansers are less damaging

For best results use products containing cocamidopropyl betaine or coco betaine.

Good Shampoo Ingredients:

- Sodium laureth sulfate: A mild cleansing agent derived from coconut oil. Used in many products for its foaming and cleansing properties. Gently removes grease from the hair and skin.
- Cocamidopropylamine Oxide: Extracted from palm nuts, it is a mild detergent with conditioning properties.
- Propylene glycole: Derived from coconut oil, it attracts and locks in moisture.
- Lauramide DEA: Derived from palm trees, it is a gentle foam enhancer.

Conditioners are used to change the texture and appearance of the hair

- Replenish moisture, body, strength, and manageability of the hair
- Replace natural oils that have been washed away by shampoo
- Deep conditioners benefit normal, dry and damaged hair
- Penetrates the cuticle

Things to know if you are going to follow a co-wash conditioner only regimen:

- Do your homework and understand silicones
- Avoid water insoluble and organic insoluble materials

- Non-water soluble build up on the hair can block out moisture
- If you are co-washing daily, use a moisturizing conditioner that is silicone-free
- For best results, use products only containing the Dimethicone Copolyols or PEG-modified dimethicones

Good Conditioner Ingredients:

- Cetheth 20: Moisturizer derived from palm oil
- Panthenol: Moisturizer and conditioning agent derived from vitamin B5
- Ceearyl alcohol: Moisturizer and thickening agent

Moisturizers are used to prevent the scalp and hair from becoming too dry

- Replenish moisture, body, strength and manageability of the hair
- Replace natural oils that have been washed away by shampoo
- Deep conditioners benefit normal, dry and damaged hair
- Penetrates the cuticle

Things to know if you are going to use a moisturizing regimen:

- All oils are sealants
- Many oils operate differently in the hair
- Seal in moisture with a non-water base product

- Raw shea butters can give a stronger hold or seal
- Some oils sit on top of the strand coating the cuticle more as a sealant for moisture
- Few oils have a molecular structure small enough to penetrate the hair shaft and induce moisture

Good Moisturizer Ingredients:

- Cetheth 20: Moisturizer derived from palm oil
- Panthenol: Moisturizer and conditioning agent derived from vitamin B5
- Ceearyl alcohol: Moisturizer and thickening agent

10 Ingredients to Avoid

Most commercially available hair care products use harmful, potentially carcinogenic ingredients. Below is a list of those that have been named the worst common product ingredients found in things you put on your hair and body. The more of a particular ingredient you have in a product, the closer it is to the top of the list of ingredients on the packaging:

- Isopropyl Alcohol
- Mineral Oil & Petrolatum Peg
- Propylene Glycol (Pg)
- Sodium Lauryl Sulfate (Sls) & Sodium Laureth Sulfate (Sles)
- Sodium Laureth Sulfate (Sles)
- Chlorine

- Dea (Diethanolamine) Mea (Momoethnanolamine) Tea Triethanolamine
- Fd & C Color Pigments
- Fragrance
- Imidazolidinvl Urea and Dmdm Hydantoin

Benefits of natural products and herbal supplements

When you make your own natural hair products you know exactly what you're getting. Do you know what you are getting in your commercial products? Did you know that if a product contains 5% of a natural substance it can be labeled 100% natural?

Due to time constraints, I personally do not make all of the products that I use in my hair. The one product that I do choose to make is my own deep conditioner.

A basic DIY deep conditioner could consist of:

- Cream based conditioner
- Cream based leave-in conditioner
- 2 to 3 natural oils
- Honey

Be creative! You could sit under a dryer or heating cap for 20 minutes or allow it to stay in your hair overnight

Benefits of buying products from small business product vendors

Most are homemade using natural ingredients. But even with small vendors and whole food stores, you should still do your research to verify that what you are getting is authentically natural.

All natural products that benefit your hair

There are several beneficial all natural products out there. Below are a few products found in some of the top all natural homemade hair products and remedies.

1. Essential oils are natural oils that are extracted from the leaves, stems, flowers or bark of a plant and benefit both your hair and scalp. Some uses are listed below:

   • Cleanses the scalp, strengthens hair, controls irritation and dandruff
   • Stimulates hair follicles, improves circulation and even promotes hair growth
   • Improves the condition of the scalp
   • Improves the condition of the hair

2. Extra virgin coconut oil is beneficial for the skin, weight loss, digestion, immune system, heart disease and even helps to fight infections. A few benefits of using coconut oil in the hair are listed below:

- Promotes strength and hair growth
- Keeps the scalp from flaking
- Keeps the hair conditioned and moisturized
- Increases the protein retention in the hair
- Often used as a remedy for hair loss

3. Extra virgin olive oil is beneficial for digestion, heart disease and promoting healthy aging. It is naturally free of cholesterol, unsaturated fat, salt, sugar and gluten, and is rich in good monounsaturated fat. A few benefits of using olive oil in the hair are shown below:

- Helps hair look healthier, stronger and shinier
- Prevents breakage, splitting and frizzy fly-aways
- Keeps ends from looking messy and unkempt
- Smooths away some of those flaking problems
- Adds weight and moisture to the hair

4. Apple cider vinegar is beneficial for weight loss, acne, sunburn, weight gain, indigestion, acid reflux, gas, hemorrhoids, infections, kidney stones, gall bladder stones, constipation and the list goes on and on. A few benefits of using apple cider vinegar in the hair are as follows:

- Restores silkiness and shine to hair
- Cleanses and exfoliates the scalp
- Removes buildup of hair products
- Promotes hair growth
- Kills bacteria and balances pH level

5. Aloe vera juice is beneficial for detoxification, as an emollient, alkalizing the body, cardiovascular health, boosting the immune system, skin, disinfectant, antibiotic, anti-microbial, germicidal, anti-bacterial, antiseptic, anti-fungal and anti-viral, reducing inflammation, weight loss and more. A few benefits of using Aloe Vera Juice in the hair are:

- Conditions coarse hair
- Helps reverse hair loss
- Removes excess moisture without making hair brittle
- Keeps hair soft to the touch
- Relieves and prevents itching

6. Honey is beneficial for beautiful skin, fights acne, controls diabetes, heart disease, promotes weight loss, boosts immune system, cures cough and sore throat, indigestion and more. A few benefits of using honey in the hair are listed below:

- Removes dead skin cells from the roots
- Cures dry, damaged and dull looking hair
- Retains moisture to get rid of dry itchy flakes on scalp
- Absorbs impurities from the pores on the skin
- Soothes and heals the scalp

7. Henna is a natural plant based body art and hair color that is beneficial for skin and hair treatments. The use of henna goes back more than 4000 years. 100% natural, paraphenylene diamine (PPD) free, gluten free, 100% vegan sulfate free and is generally safe for the

whole family. A few benefits of using henna in the hair are below:

- Shines, softens and conditions the hair
- Colors hair naturally and permanently
- Aids in the cure of dandruff, head lice and ringworm
- Stops splits ends and hair breakage
- Bonds to proteins in the hair

My 12 basic "go-to" products

I have listed my 12 basic "go-to" products to give you an idea of how to put together products for your own regimen. I did not name the brands because it is important for you to determine what brands work best for your hair.

1. Extra Virgin Vinegar – to exfoliate the scalp
2. Honey – in my deep conditioner for shine
3. Cholesterol conditioner – to create my deep conditioner recipe
4. Conditioner leave-in – spray
5. Conditioner leave-in – cream
6. Conditioner henna – to condition, color and naturally stretch my hair
7. Oils – to pre-rinse for moisture seal
8. Spray moisturizer – for my braids, twists and coils
9. Activator gel – for moisturizing
10. Styling gel – for setting styles
11. Serum – for flat ironing or hot pressing

12. Clarifying shampoo – to strip occasional build up, residue of salt water or chlorine from swimming

Create your 12 basic "go-to" products list

Creating your personal "go-to" product list is one of the first things that I would suggest you get started on as a natural. If you are transitioning on your own or with a stylist, you may find that some of the products that your hair loves now will continue to work on your journey. You just need to make sure the ingredients in them are good for you. My bestie, (in my head), Curly Nikki, has done an amazing job assisting naturals in finding great products for their hair. In her book, *Better than Good Hair* by Nikki Walton, she has a very helpful Comprehensive Natural Hair Product Guide full of cleansers, conditioners, oils, sealants and stylers. It even comes with a key to show you which products are non-sulfate, how to save money and much more. Check it out!

As you move forward, you should begin to find and choose your own "go-to" products. Make a list and remember some of the products on your list could change a few times before you nail down what is truly right for you.

1.

2.

3.

4.

5.

6.

7.

8.

9.

10.

11.

12.

CHAPTER THREE

USE PROPER HAIR TOOLS AND TECHNIQUES

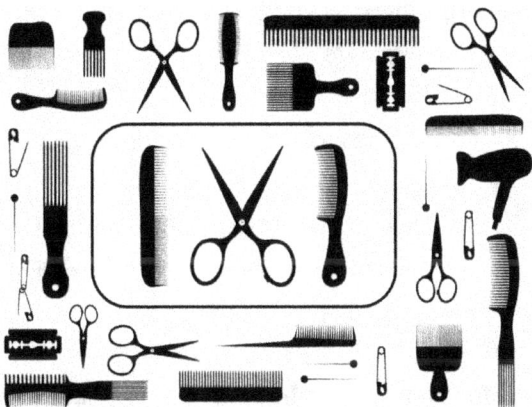

Use proper hair tools and techniques

Using the proper tools in caring for your hair is important. What you decide to put in your tool kit will be based on what will work for you at each stage. The following are tools that are good to consider having in your hair arsenal.

Hair care tools

Applicator bottles – to apply liquid or cream-based products

Applicator brush – to evenly apply creamy textured products like conditioners, colors, texturizers or relaxers to the hair

Bobby pins (big/small), hairpins and spiral pins – work easily for securing buns and updos

Bonnet and pillowcase (silk or satin) – to protect the hair from drying out overnight

Bowls – for holding tools and mixing products

Brush for styling (Denman, wig, paddle) – popular brushes used for detangling wet or dry, natural and relaxed hair

Brush for waves (medium bristle) – lays down and smooths waves with soft, medium or heavy bristles

Containers – to store hair products or items

Curlformers, large rollers (roller papers) – to set the hair in curls

Funnel – transfer liquid from one container to another

Gloves – to protect the hands from residue or other products that could cause a mess when doing the hair

Hair bands – these will hold the hair in sections and prevent hair from unraveling or falling. Mostly used to put the hair in a ponytail

Hair clips, pins and claws (large/small) – for strong hold on updos and pin ups

Hair shears – to trim the hair and cut off split ends

Hand blow dryer with diffuser – to dry curly hair without disturbing the curls and for smooth blowouts

Handheld mirror – to see the back of your head when styling your hair

Hooded dryer – gives a professional salon look to your styles and locks in conditioners and moisture

Microfiber towels (T-shirts) – to dry the hair without pulling or snagging the strands

Paddle brush – for detangling and smoothing natural or relaxed hair

Rat tail comb – good for parting and sectioning

Scarfs, stocking caps and du-rags – to protect the hair from the elements, under wigs and while sleeping

Spray bottles – to apply water and moisturizers to hair

Toothbrush (soft) – to slick and smooth straight or wavy edges

Wide tooth comb – to detangle hair and minimize hair loss when used on wet or dry curly hair

Sectioning hair for regimens and techniques

You can expect to be better able to manipulate your hair if you handle the hair in sections. The sections do not have to be perfect. Use any type of hair clips to section the hair prior to any regimen or styling to keep down shedding. The number of sections you use to do this should be based on the length and thickness of your hair.

- 2 sections – 1 in the front and back or 1 on each side
- 4 sections – 2 in the front and 2 in the back
- 5 sections – 2 in the front, 1 in the top middle, 2 in the back
- 6 sections – 2 in the front, 1 in the middle, 3 in the back or 3 on each side)
- 10 or more sections – 5 on each side

Coach's Tip: You can also twist or put your hair in plaits to cleanse or color the hair in sections. The hair acts like a sponge and the shampoo, color or conditioners will penetrate it. If you decide to go this route, make sure that you do a thorough rinse so that you don't leave any product residue in your hair.

Finger detangling, combing and palm brushing

Dry Detangling

Dry detangling is great for naturals who tangle easily or who are about to shampoo their hair. This is done by applying oil, conditioner or a mixture of the two to the hair, and detangling it before you cleanse. For best results, allow the product to absorb into the hair overnight. This method works for several reasons:

- It can be done in front of the mirror and out of the shower to make it easier to see and remove the tangles.
- There is less chance for breakage since the hair is strongest when dry.
- The oils and/or conditioners not only act as a lubricant for easier detangling, but they also help to moisturize the hair to reduce the dryness and matting that shampooing can cause.

Wet Detangling

Wet detangling involves detangling the hair when it is wet and well lubricated with a conditioner that has good slip. Slip is moisture saturation that causes dry or tangled hair to unravel with ease. The reasons why this method is so well loved are because:

- When the hair is wet it is more elastic and it is easier to detangle.
- The conditioner and the water create more slip than oil and conditioner.

Tips for detangling your hair wet or dry

- Use a conditioner or moistening product that has slip
- Separate the hair at the roots horizontally to loosen it
- Remove hair that has shed as you go through your hair
- Gently finger-comb from end to root
- Optional: Use a wide tooth comb or Denman brush
- Look and feel for knots as you detangle your hair
- Dilute a slippery conditioner in a dye applicator bottle with water

Coach's Tips:

To remove the knots

- Saturate the knot with conditioner
- Gently separate the hair
- Do not tug or pull in a downward motion
- Do not attempt to brush or comb out knots
- Use the tip of a comb or pin to widen a tight knot

- Slide the knot up and down to release it
- Cut off knots that can't be removed
- Apply conditioner directly to knots, massage and remove strands from the core to release

Finger combing and palm brushing

- Finger combing is as simple as taking your fingers and gently raking through your hair strands.
- Palm brushing is simply taking the palms of your hands to smooth and slick down your hair.
- Taking a section of your curly hair into your hand and squeezing it while pushing it up towards your head is called scrunching.

Coach's Tip: For best results, do both. Dry detangle before a wash or co-wash with oil or moisturizer. This can reduce a lot of shedding when detangling wet hair during or after cleansing with a conditioner.

My grandmother told me that we shed 1000 strands of hair a day. I decided I would do some research on this. Here is what I found.

According to the Griffin Center for hair restoration and research, the average person sheds around 100 telogen-stage hairs a day between brushing, showering and other activities. *Telogen* is the name for the resting stage of the hair growth cycle. High-stress and trauma like high fevers, nutritional deficiencies, pneumonia and accidents can cause hair to shed in higher than normal amounts.

Dr. Susan C. Taylor, a Harvard trained dermatologist, clinical researcher and world-renowned expert in treating skin of color for over 20 years stated in the Huffington post, "The hair of many black women is very fragile and studies have demonstrated that normal brushing and combing of the hair can result in breakage. Brushing your hair 100 times a day is a no-no for black hair. It is recommended that you comb and brush your hair only to style it."

To control frizz

- You can wet hair and apply conditioner daily
- Rinse hair in cool water after a wash or co-wash

NOTES:

_____

_____

_____

_____

CHAPTER FOUR

HEALTHY HAIR BASIC REGIMENS

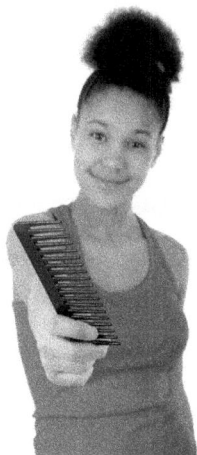

Basic "how to" regimens for textured,
processed or transitioning hair

Transforming to your natural good hair requires taming your hair to effectively respond to regular maintenance. This includes keeping your hair clean, conditioned, moisturized and trimmed. Establishing a hair regimen means that you will set aside specific times to be consistent in practicing healthy hair care that is specific to your hair type and desired style. After a while you should be able to master the basic steps and become more creative. The following regimens are not set in stone, so please feel free to use the section provided at the end of each regimen to write notes and make them your own. In this section you will find the basic steps on how to do the following:

- Pre-poo
- Oil rinse
- Co-wash
- Exfoliate scalp
- Shampoo wash
- Condition
- Deep condition
- LOC in moisture
- Define curl pattern
- Blow out natural hair
- Trim textured or curly hair
- Trim straight hair
- Sleep on your hair
- Work out with your hair
- Swim with your hair

Coach's Tip: *Never* scrub products into your hair as this could cause tangles and knots. You should separate the hair into 4 or more sections for most of the following regimens. However, straight or relaxed hair may only need 2 to 3 sections. Below are a few drying tips for those wet regimens:

Drying Tips

- Wrapping the hair with a microfiber towel or T-shirt helps the hair to dry faster
- Hood dry curly or straight hair on warm, low or cool to avoid damage
- Blow dry curly or straight hair on warm, low or cool to avoid damage
- Blow dry straight hair using a diffuser to create volume or waves
- Blow dry curly hair using a diffuser to avoid frizzing
- Blow or hood dry curly hair about 80% and then allow hair to air dry
- *Do not* manipulate curly hair while it is drying, you may cause frizz
- Scrunch curly hair with a microfiber towel or T-shirt to remove excess water

How to pre-poo

During the normal washing process your hair soaks up water and swells. As the water escapes it also takes some of the moisture and protein from your hair. Your hair strands then contract to their normal size and are weak and prone to breakage.

Pre-pooing with oil is a very effective method for combating the negative effects of washing your hair. When you pre-poo, the hair strands are coated with oil, strengthening them and preventing them from soaking in too much water.

What you will need:

- Oil moisturizer
- Plastic cap
- Towel
- Head wrap
- Wide tooth comb (optional)
- Hair clips
- Applicator bottle
- Spray bottle

Follow these steps:

- Section hair into 4 to 6 sections
- Work on one section at a time
- Apply water to each section
- Separate hair within the section
- Saturate with oil from root to tip
- Twist the section
- Apply plastic cap
- Allow heat penetration overnight, then let sit for 30 minutes or sit under dryer 20 minutes
- Finger comb and detangle each section (wide tooth comb is optional)
- Twist the section
- Co-wash or wash as usual

Coach's Tip: *Do not* use conditioners to pre-poo the hair. Only a few oils can penetrate hair strands, causing less breakage. Coconut oil is an oil that I use to stop my hair from absorbing too much water during the wash. It will also protect the hair from protein loss and dehydration.

NOTES:

_____

_____

_____

_____

How to oil rinse

Oil rinsing is similar to the pre-poo routine. The purpose of the oil rinse is to keep your hair strands strong while adding shine and gloss.

What you will need:

- Oil sealant
- Plastic cap
- Towel
- Head wrap
- Wide tooth comb (optional)
- Hair clips
- Applicator bottle
- Water spray bottle

Follow these steps:

1. Work on one section at a time
2. Separate hair within the section
3. Saturate with oil from root to tip
4. Finger comb and detangle
5. Twist the section
6. Put on plastic cap
7. Allow heat penetration for 10 minutes or sit under dryer 20 minutes
8. Wet hair and smooth through
9. Reapply oil and rinse again
10. Twist the section
11. Co-wash out excess oil
12. Style as usual

Coach's Tip: After applying oil, you don't have to use conditioner. The hair will be as smooth as it is after applying regular conditioner. This is also a great way to define your curl pattern.

NOTES:

_____

_____

_____

_____

How to co-wash

The curly girl method is a popular way to cleanse curly hair without shampoo. The process can be found in the *Curly Girl Handbook*, which was written by Lorraine Massey. The no poo method described in her book helps to keep from stripping the hair of its natural oils. Many naturals have modified the CG method (using light silicones, straightening hair with a flat iron, clarifying with a sulfate free shampoo, etc.) because it works for them. The modified process described here is using conditioner in place of shampoo to cleanse and moisturize the hair, light oil to seal in moisture and a light gel, mousse or setting lotion to hold your style. This was designed to be a basic guideline to assist you in creating a regimen that works for you. Create a routine where you choose a day to co-wash. This can be done once a week, bi-weekly or monthly depending on what type of style you are wearing. You can also refresh your co-wash weekly or as needed. It is recommended that you give your hair 2 – 4 weeks to adjust to the no poo cleansing method.

What you will need:

- Conditioner cleanser
- Conditioner leave in (liquid or cream)
- Oil moisturizer
- Hair gel or mousse or setting lotion
- Applicator bottle
- Spray bottle with water
- Wide tooth comb
- Hair clips

- Microfiber towel or old T-Shirt
- Optional: Extra Virgin Vinegar

Follow these steps:

1. Optional: Pre-poo the night before or one hour prior to co-wash
2. Section hair into 4 to 6 sections
3. Work on one section at a time
4. Apply co-wash conditioner to saturate the hair starting at the ends
5. Massage to cleanse the scalp with the conditioner
6. Separate and detangle the section
7. Rinse while finger combing the section
8. Squeeze out excess water
9. Optional: Apply oil sealant
10. Apply cream leave-in conditioner
11. Clip or twist the section
12. Continue to the next section until complete
13. Wrap head with microfiber towel or T-shirt (plopping) to absorb excess water
14. Style as usual

Coach's Tip: To refresh your co-wash, complete the same regimen using a spray bottle to apply water to start the process on damp or dry hair. According to the curly girl method, a final rinse of your hair with cool or cold water will decrease frizz and add shine. Try that if you'd like.

NOTES:

_____

_____

_____

_____

How to exfoliate scalp

What you will need:

- Apple Cider Vinegar
- Applicator bottle
- Spray bottle containing water
- Microfiber towel or old T-Shirt
- Optional: Wide tooth comb
- Hair clips

Follow these steps:

1. Section hair into 4 to 6 sections
2. Work through one section at a time
3. Mix 1 cup of apple cider vinegar to 2 cups of water
4. Optional: Add a drop of your favorite essential oil
5. Apply mixed solution to scalp
6. Hold the end of hair and scrub on scalp with pads of fingers

7. Finger comb and rinse thoroughly
8. Twist or clip that section and continue to the next
9. Rinse thoroughly
10. Optional: Move on to the co-wash regimen

Coach's Tip: An essential oil is a concentrated hydrophobic liquid containing volatile aroma compounds from plants. Some of the best penetrating essential oils are coconut, olive and grape seed. To cleanse your hair tools, soak them overnight in the same mixed vinegar and water solution.

NOTES:

_____

_____

_____

_____

How to shampoo wash

In order to cleanse your hair of any silicones, you must clarify with a sulfate shampoo. This will deep cleanse and strip build up from the hair.

What you will need:

• Clarifying shampoo (to strip build up)

- Optional: Moisturizing shampoo
- Optional: Extra Virgin Vinegar (to exfoliate the scalp)
- Conditioner cleanser
- Leave-in conditioner (liquid or cream)
- Oil moisturizer
- Applicator bottle
- Spray bottle
- Microfiber towel or old T-Shirt
- Optional: Wide tooth comb
- Hair clips

Follow these steps:

1. Section hair into 4 to 6 sections
2. Work on one section at a time
3. Apply shampoo to wet hair starting at the ends
4. Hold the end of hair and scrub shampoo on scalp with pad of finger
5. Finger comb and rinse thoroughly
6. Twist that section and continue to the next
7. Optional: Apply oil moisturizer and finger detangle
8. Apply leave-in conditioner and finger detangle
9. Twist the section and go to the next
10. Wrap with microfiber towel or T-shirt (plopping) to absorb excess water
11. Style as usual

Coach's Tip: For your "wash and go," do not touch hair while it is drying. This helps to avoid altering your style or causing frizz. Scrunch gently to remove stiffness after hair is completely dry.

NOTES:

_____

_____

_____

_____

How to condition

What you will need:

- Conditioner
- Spray bottle containing water

Follow these steps:

1. Start on clean, damp hair
2. Optional: Dampen hair with spray bottle
3. Divide into 4 to 6 sections
4. Finger comb and detangle
5. Clip or twist each section
6. Apply conditioner to each section
7. Twist hair sections as you go
8. Apply plastic cap and scarf
9. Optional: Sit under dryer for 15 to 20 minutes
10. Rinse out each twist
11. Oil and re-twist each section as you go

12. Wrap with microfiber towel of T-shirt (Plopping) to absorb excess water
13. Scrunch gently to avoid altering your pattern or causing frizz
14. Style as usual

Coach's Tip: Deep condition at least once a month or as often as needed. Henna is also a great natural conditioner.

NOTES:

_____

_____

_____

_____

How to deep condition

What you will need:

- Creamy conditioner
- Scalp oil
- Raw coconut oil
- Honey
- Your favorite hair oil
- Old T-Shirt to dry hair

- Applicator brush

Follow these steps:

1. Mix 1 cup conditioner, 1 tbsp. of honey and 1 tbsp. hair oil in a bowl
2. Stir to creamy consistency
3. Pour into applicator bottle
4. Start on clean damp hair and divide hair into 4 to 6 sections
5. Finger comb and detangle
6. Clip or twist hair
7. Apply conditioner evenly with applicator bottle or brush
8. Twist hair sections as you go
9. Apply plastic cap, Saran wrap and scarf
10. Exercise, sit under dryer 1 hour or leave on overnight
11. Shampoo or co-wash and condition
12. Rinse out each twist, oil and re-twist
13. Wrap with microfiber towel or t-shirt (plopping) to absorb excess water
14. Scrunch gently to avoid altering your pattern or causing frizz
15. Style as usual

Coach's Tip: Deep condition once a week to train your hair for a healthy transformation. Once you feel the time is right, you can then begin deep conditioning once a month. Henna is also a great natural conditioner.

NOTES:

_____

_____

_____

_____

How to loc in moisture

I mentioned in Chapter 2 how most naturals struggle with dry hair syndrome (DHS). Before we move forward, I think it is important that you know how to loc in and retain the moisture in your hair.

The biggest mistakes we make as naturals is piling on products. If "they" say it works for dry hair, thinning hair or growing the hair, then most of us will run to get it and try it. Well keep in mind that "they" don't know your hair like you do. It's not always about the products; it is more about the methods used to get the products to work.

First things first, STOP applying products to your dry hair! Have you ever tried applying dish washing liquid to a dry sponge? Uh yeah, it's just lying on the sponge just like that product is just lying on your hair. Your natural hair is like that sponge. I can prove it. Wet it and see if it doesn't swell up and become heavy with water. Once it is wet take your hand and squeeze it and see if the water doesn't run out of it the same way it does from a sponge.

You want to always apply product to wet or damp hair and squeeze it into the hair so it does not end up just sitting on top of the hair. Once that product is in the hair, you want it to stay in the hair, right? Well, the last step would be to seal it into the hair with a sealant product.

If this is the first time you have heard of this process, know that it is not new, just new to you. What I have just described is a process affectionately known as the LOC method in the curly hair community. Although, it has been modified by some naturals to benefit us more, it stills works just the same.

The LOC method is simply layering the products on the hair for moisture retention. This process generally works best for thicker hair types. If you have thin dry hair, take precaution when using this method. Too much product can cause thinner hair to limp. Now, make this a part of your regular routine and struggle with dry hair no more!

What you will need:

- Applicator bottle
- Spray bottle containing water
- Leave-in conditioner (liquid)
- Oil Moisturizer
- Cream based moisturizer (i.e. butters, leave in conditioner)
- Microfiber towel or old T-Shirt
- Optional: Wide tooth comb
- Hair clips

Follow these steps:

1. Start with damp washed or co-washed hair
2. Section and twist or clip hair
3. Take down a section and spray water
4. Optional: Mix water with leave-in conditioner
5. Add oil moisture of your choice to each section
6. Add cream-based curl enhancer of your choice (butters, leave-in conditioners) to seal in the oil
7. Separate and smooth ½ inch or 1inch pieces of hair with curl enhancer
8. Air dry or sit under dryer
9. Do not touch hair while drying to avoid altering curl pattern or causing frizz
10. Scrunch gently to remove any stiffness after hair is completely dry
11. Style as usual

Coach's Tip: ALWAYS hydrate your hair with water to prepare it for products. For the best results, test your hair's porosity prior to using the LOC method. This way you can be sure that you are using products that will work for your hair. Remember to use the LOC method prior to doing techniques where you want to retain moisture for your styles.

NOTES:

_____

_____

How to define curls

Getting the hair to curl during the transition process is a little difficult, but once you are completely natural you will experience better results when defining your curl pattern. To get your strands to naturally curl, you must train them using the right tools, techniques and products.

Keep the hair moisturized so that it will do what it should naturally do, which is to coil, curl or wave. Your hair could be dry for several reasons. But in many cases, products that are not compatible for your type and texture can cause hair to lose its natural hydration.

The most important part of defining your curl pattern is creating the clump. That's right, the clump. I know it sounds strange, but the clump that you feel is the actual curl in the hair. Be careful though, because some of them could become knots, and that is why detangling your hair the right way is important. Follow the detangle regimen in Chapter 4.

Curl defining will always start with regular washing or co-washing, moisturizing and deep conditioning. You can train your hair with twists, braids, Bantu knots, shingling, curl clumping, curl sets and wash and go's. If you can master finger combing, palm brushing and scrunching, your curls should last longer.

What you will need:

- Optional: Clarifying shampoo (to strip build up)
- Optional: Extra Virgin Vinegar
- Applicator bottle
- Spray bottle containing water
- Conditioner cleanser
- Leave-in conditioner (liquid or cream)
- Oil moisturizer
- Microfiber towel or old T-Shirt
- Optional: Wide tooth comb
- Hair clips

Follow these steps:

1. Start with damp washed or co-washed hair
2. Section and twist or clip hair
3. Take down a section and add leave-in conditioner
4. Optional: Add moisture of your choice to each section
5. Add curl enhancer of your choice (gel, mousse, setting lotion)
6. Optional: Shingling - Separate and smooth ½ inch or 1inch pieces of hair with curl enhancer
7. Optional: Twist, braid, Bantu knot - Separate, braid or twist with curl enhancer
8. Optional: Wrap or pin roots if you want them to lay down smoothly
9. Air dry or sit under dryer
10. Do not touch hair while drying to avoid altering curl pattern or causing frizz

11. Scrunch gently to remove stiffness after hair is completely dry

12. Style as usual

Coach's Tip: It is recommended that you follow this process a few times and wear it for at least 3 to 5 days to train your curl pattern. If you want to blow dry the hair, hold a diffuser dryer close to your head on cool or medium setting. Scrunch to remove stiffness after the hair is completely dry.

NOTES:

_____

_____

_____

_____

How to blow out

What you will need:

- Deep conditioner
- Leave-in conditioner
- Oil

- Serum
- Paddle brush
- Silk scarf
- Blow dryer (handheld)

Follow these steps:

1. Co-wash
2. Deep condition if needed
3. Divide into 4 to 6 sections
4. Apply leave-in conditioner
5. Add blow drying cream or serum as you go through
6. Begin blowing out each section using the tension method (hold the hair on the ends while moving the dryer up and down the hair strands)
7. Apply oil or non-water-based product for shine
8. Use paddle brush to smooth and detangle blown out hair with blow dryer on low setting
9. Use warm air to dry (or cool air, but it takes longer)

Coach's Tip: Use smaller sections if your hair is thicker. Blow dry your hair on low temperature to avoid heat damage.

NOTES:

_____

_____

_____

How to quick trim

If you find that your hair consistently tangles, it may be time for a trim. Sometimes getting rid of damaged hair will make it easier to manage. If you don't have a regular stylist to do it for you, you can always quick trim it yourself.

Trim Textured or Curly Hair

What you will need:

- Hair scissors
- Ponytail holder
- Towel or T-shirt

Follow these steps:

- Wash or co-wash
- Detangle
- Add medium size twists to damp hair
- Let hair dry completely
- Option 1: Unravel dry twist at the ends (about an inch). Clip the ends of each individual twist
- Option 2: Unravel to a twist out and clip ends that are transparent

Coach's Tip:

- Avoid trimming curly hair when it is wet. Curly hair expands when it is wet and shrinks when it is dry, so you may trim too much if it is wet.
- Trim textured hair every six to eight months about a quarter inch.

NOTES:

_____

_____

_____

_____

Trim straight hair

What you will need:

- Hair scissors
- Scrunchy
- Towel or T-shirt

Follow these steps:

1. Put the hair in one high ponytail (for layers) or two low side ponytails

2. Close the end of the ponytail with another scrunchy or ponytail hair band
3. Trim or cut the ends

Coach's Tip:

*   It is recommended that you trim straight hair while it is wet to avoid taking off too much of your length.
*   If your hair is going to revert back to its curly texture with water, then you can trim the hair while it is dry.
*   Less than a quarter inch is a trim. Any more than that is a cut.

NOTES:

_____

_____

_____

_____

How to protect your hair while working out

Protecting your hair during your workout is important so you don't sweat out the moisture in your hair.

What you will need:

- Scrunchy
- Brush for straightening
- Scarf or mesh wrap

Follow these steps:

1. Pull hair up into a high ponytail
2. Secure with hair scrunchy
3. Lay scarf or mesh wrap around the edges of the hair (optional for textured or curly hair)

Coach's Tip: If the hair is straight, remove the scarf about an hour later to make sure that your roots and edges are dry underneath. If your hair is textured or curly, you can remove the scarf immediately after the workout is complete. Use the same routine to avoid wet edges from the steam of a shower. Washing the hair after a workout is optional, but not recommended unless it is absolutely necessary.

NOTES:

_____

_____

_____

_____

How to prepare your hair for swimming

What you will need:

- Spray bottle with water
- Conditioner (inexpensive and natural)
- Oil

Follow these steps:

1. Spray hair with water
2. Separate hair into 4 sections
3. Saturate the hair with water and work it through
4. Coat every strand of the section with conditioner
5. Coat every strand of the section with oil
6. Twist the section, pull up into a bun and go
7. Optional: Lycra or spandex cap for additional protection
8. Optional: Add a silicone swim cap on top of that, if you're real skeeeerd!

Coach's Tip: White coating from the product will go away shortly after applying. After swimming, do a quick co-wash and go. You could also make 6 to 8 braids to make the detangling process easier later.

NOTES:

_____

_____

_____

How to sleep on your natural hair

What you will need:

* Silk or satin pillowcase
* Silk or satin scarf

Follow these steps:

To protect your hair while sleeping, it is recommended that you sleep on a satin pillowcase with your hair pulled up into a high ponytail on the top of your head (also known as the pineapple). Cover the hair with a silk scarf or bonnet.

Coach's Tip: You can also use a wrap to secure the hair in place. Follow the same instructions when napping to preserve your style and reduce frizz.

NOTES:

_____

_____

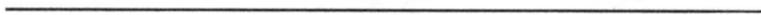

CHAPTER FIVE

MASTER BASIC HAIR TECHNIQUES

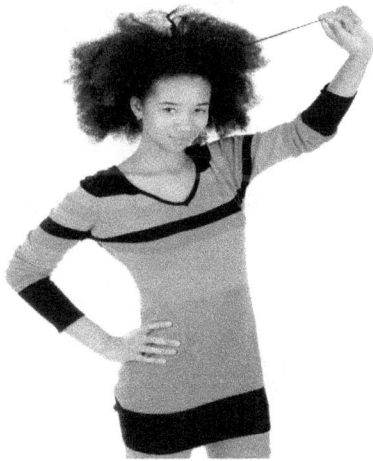

Eight basic "how to" techniques for transition and protective styles

One of the challenges with ethnic hair among women is that every woman wants to look her best at every stage in the game. It doesn't matter if you are transitioning, textured or wearing straight hair. Mastering basic styling techniques is important for achieving that professional, fresh out of the salon look. In this section you will find basics steps on how to:

- Find your "go to" protective or transition style
- Properly twist or braid for styling
- Wet set natural or straight hair
- Quick set curly or straight hair
- Flat iron curly or straight hair
- Create waves or curls on short to medium hair
- Stretch natural hair for length
- Create the deep wave bun
- Taper your straight or wavy edges
- Care for your braids, twists and dreadlocks

How to properly twist and braid for styling

Braiding and twisting will be used for several protective and transitional styles. These are all both great ways to train your natural hair's curl definition. Many naturals agree these are also good ways to stretch your hair out for more length. Although we touched on how to define your curls in another chapter, I thought it was important to discuss the proper techniques here.

One of the things I never hear talked about in the natural hair care industry is the proper way to secure braids and twists. As much as we use these techniques to style and maintain our hair, it is important to know how to properly secure these styles without causing damage to the scalp. When you secure your hair properly it will also allow for an easier take down. This will save time and unwanted damage to your hair strands.

First things first, *do not* twist or braid your hair too tight. The process itself is going to secure the style and keep the hair from unraveling. There is no reason for your hair to be tight. Pulling too tight on the hair can cause hair loss and scalp damage.

When separating the hair into small sections to begin a braid or twist, section the hair as evenly as possible. The most important thing to remember is: *do not* re-split the hair while braiding or twisting even when adding extensions to the hair.

What is Re-Splitting?

Re-splitting happens when you are braiding or twisting the hair and, as you are going down, you start taking hair from each strand to even the hair out as you braid down the hair. When re-splitting the hair you can cause more knotting and tangling during the takedown process. If you must re-split the hair, it is best to do it at the end of the braid or twist. This way it will be easier to find the starting point during the takedown. That way you won't get tangles and knots in the middle or at the roots during the process.

Coach's Tip: It is important to hold your hands in the correct position when braiding or twisting the hair; be sure to hold your thumbs in an upright position throughout the process. This will allow you to control the strands for a neat, secure finish without pulling to make the hair tight. This can also help to avoid aching or the development of carpal tunnel in your hands.

Find your "go to" protective or transition style

What is a protective style?

A protective style encloses the ends of the hair to protect it from damage caused by the sun, the wind and friction. A good "go to" protective style will maintain your healthy ends and preserve your length, which will promote hair growth.

The benefits of wearing a protective style are to lock in moisture, protect the ends and retain length. If you are transitioning, protective styles will allow you to protect the new growth from breaking while the hair is growing out.

What is a "go to" style?

A "go to" style gives your tresses a break from the everyday stress of hair maintenance and frequent manipulation. A "go to" style requires less manipulation of the strands and can also be a protective style if it contributes to the hair retaining moisture and being healthy.

There are three types of "go to" styles: natural, extensions and wigs.

Natural style options allow you to wash or co-wash regularly. The styles can be re-done daily or be set for 5 to 7 days of wear. Natural styles use your hair only. Wash and go curls, twists, braid outs and buns are a few beneficial styles that we will discuss more in detail.

Extension style options can give the hair 6 to 8 weeks of rest from manipulation of the strands. Most extensions allow for a variety of style options. It is important to match texture and color for a more natural and realistic look. Braids, sew-ins and crochet are a few beneficial options for transitioning and protecting the hair.

Wig styles are great for securing long-term styles. Wig styles give you a variety of options. This is a great way to test various hair colors and determine looks that work best for you. Human and synthetic hair options are available for full and half wigs.

My favorite "protective" style is my deep wave bun, and my "go to" style is my signature Q'coil style. I tend to fluctuate between the two. The deep wave bun allows me to co-wash and set my bun weekly and wear it for 5 to 7 days (two weeks if I sleep on my face for a few days, ha ha). I like the Q'coils because I don't have to add extensions to my hair; I can style, color, co-wash and wear them for up to 8 weeks with a good hair care regimen. This style also allows me to wear a wig on occasion to change up my look. I can be just as versatile when I am wearing my braids and twists also.

I can't say what your style should be, but it should make you feel confident and free. First determine what your hair needs, find your "go to" protective style and rock it!

Avoid These 16 "Go To" Transition and Protective Style Mistakes

1. Blow drying too often – Can cause breakage and extra drying of the scalp

    Option: Occasionally use a hooded dryer or air dry regularly instead.

2. Shampooing too often – Can strip the hair of its natural oils and cause dry scalp

    Option: Shampoo less (or no more) and opt to use the co-wash regimen.

3. Styling too often – Can cause stress on the strands from constant manipulation

    Option: Give it a break! Wear styles that last longer.

4. Drying with a towel - Can pull at the strands of wet hair causing them to break

    Option: Use a microfiber towel or T-shirt to squeeze, scrunch or plop excess moisture.

5. Pulling hair too tight – Can cause permanent damage to the scalp and stop hair growth

    Option: Loosen up! The style will still last and look just as nice.

6. Causing friction – Is another way to damage and loose hair strands

   Option: Wrap it up! Your hair, I mean. The hair strands won't rub up against your clothes, jewelry or linen while you sleep.

7. Always touching your hair – Can also cause friction

   Option: Use a "Go To" style for a while and leave it alone. Find a look that you love and just wear it.

8. Using improper tools – Can pull and tug at the hair the wrong way and cause damage

   Option: Learn what tools work best for your hair.

9. Securing styles incorrectly - Can cause knotting and breakage during the take down process

   Option: Secure your styles the right way for an easier take down

10. Becoming a product junkie – Can cost you a lot of money over time

    Option: Find products that work well with your hair and stick with them. If it's not broken don't try to fix it! Have a swap party to get rid of the products that don't work for you.

11. Combing, brushing and manipulating dry hair - Can cause breakage and frizz

    Option: Keep a spray bottle of water near to mist or dampen your hair prior to handling it.

12. Coating hair with too much product - Can cause product to build up and lie on top of the strands

    Option: Mist or Dampen the hair prior to adding product, so that you don't end up using too much.

13. Following bad hair regimens - Can cause issues if they are not designed to benefit your hair type and texture.

    Option: Tweak regimens that don't work for your hair. Add your own spin to make them your own.

14. Being too cheap - Can leave you using products that will not work for your hair.

    Option: If your hair responds to an expensive brand, use it. Look for sales and coupons to keep it in your mix.

15. Too much direct heat or wind - Can cause damage during season changes

    Option: Occasionally wear head wraps and hats to protect hair from inclement weather.

16. Inexperienced hairstylist - Can do things to your hair that cause more damage

Option: Know your own hair! Take control and educate your stylist about your individual hair needs.

How to wet and dry set styles on curly or straight hair

The two ways to set natural and straight hair are wet set or dry set. It is not good to apply a lot of product to the hair for styling, but if you must, use a holding product to set your hair. Keep in mind that thin hair will usually respond better to a light holding product, such as leave-in conditioner or mousse. Thicker hair will respond better with medium to heavy holding products, such as gels or setting lotions.

How to Wet Set Natural or Straight Hairstyles Curl Set on Curly or Straight Hair

What you will need:

- Leave-in cream conditioner, gel or setting lotion
- Rollers, perm rods, drinking straws or curlformers (36+ curlers based on thickness of hair)
- End papers
- Optional: Bobby pins

Follow these steps:

1. Start on clean, wet and conditioned hair
2. Apply conditioner, gel or setting lotion on each piece of hair
3. Optional: Curlformers, flexi rods, perm rods or rollers of your choice
4. Fold end papers over the tips of hair
5. Wrap hair around curler lengthwise into spiral formation; start at the ends and roll towards the scalp
6. Secure by placing a bobby pin inside the base of the roller lengthwise at the scalp
7. Dry hair under hooded dryer until completely dry (for salon finish)
8. Optional: Air dry or dry overnight
9. Release by carefully unwinding the curler from the hair
10. Apply light oil and separate curls for more volume

Coach's Tips:

- Choose the hard plastic rollers for resistant roots
- Sponge rollers can dry out the hair (without end papers)
- Use the right setting products to limit drying time
- Sit under a warm hooded dryer if you want to quick dry
- Be sure the dryer is not too hot
- Allow approximately 6 to 8 hours to air dry
- Allow approximately 45 minutes to 1 hour to sit under the dryer

NOTES:

_____

_____

_____

_____

How to quick set natural or straight hairstyles

In a hurry? Well, here are three quick ways to set your hair on the go.

Quick Curl Set On Natural Hair

What you will need:

- Mousse or holding product
- Scarf

Follow these steps:

1. Starting on wet or dry hair, add light gel, mousse or holding product
2. Brush hair to the top of head
3. Braid or twist

4. Optional: Make two or more braids, twists or bantu knots at the top of your head
5. Taper and smooth edges
6. Wrap with scarf to dry overnight or sit under dryer

Coach's Tip: Use this simple option for a quick braid or twist-out set.

NOTES:

_____

_____

_____

_____

Quick Curl Set On Straight Hair

What you will need:

- Brush
- Mousse or holding product
- Scarf

Follow these steps:

1. Starting on dry hair, brush hair into a high ponytail on top of head
2. Add moisture to ends

3. Optional: Add a light holding product
4. Roll hair (sponge or other) use papers
5. Taper and smooth edges
6. Wrap scarf overnight (dampen ends if under dryer)

Coach's Tip: This technique works best on dry straight hair.

NOTES:

_____

_____

_____

_____

Quick Wrap set on curly or straight hair

What you will need:

- Hair pins
- Wave brush
- Scarf or wave cap
- Spray water bottle

Follow these steps:

1. Apply leave in conditioner from the ends of the hair to the root
2. Apply your favorite oil
3. Optional: Prepare a front part
4. Separate hair into two sections
5. Keep hair moist with spray water bottle
6. Brush hair flat as you wrap it around your head and add bobby pins
7. Continue adding bobby pins all around the head as you lay the hair down
8. Wrap with scarf or wave cap

Coach's Tip: You can use this technique on wet or dry hair.

NOTES:

_____

_____

_____

_____

How to create waves or curls on short to medium hair

What you will need:

- Spray bottle containing water
- Leave-in conditioner

- Holding gel
- Optional: Moisturizing gel
- Optional: Oil
- Optional: Curl enhancing product or styling treatment
- Optional: Blow dryer with diffuser

Follow these steps:

1. Start with clean, damp hair and add your leave-in conditioner of choice
2. Squeeze the product into your hair
3. Optional: Add a curl enhancing product from roots to ends
4. Optional: Add oil and/or gels
5. Finger coil or sponge brush coils into hair
6. Optional: On sections that are longer, use a brush to curl hair
7. Allow hair to air dry

Coach's Tip: When using a diffuser, start at the roots first and move in a slow circular motion. To add volume, hold dryer against the head at a 90-degree angle or flip your head upside down for about a minute. It is recommended that you use a low speed and high heat for best results. You can determine what is best for your hair.

NOTES:

_____

_____

How to stretch curly hair for length

There are several different ways that you can stretch natural hair for length. You can do this with or without heat. I will talk about three ways to stretch the hair. These options will give you the basics and allow you to be creative in coming up with options for stretching your hair in the future.

Stretch Curly Hair with Braids

What you will need:

- Spray bottle containing water
- Oil and/or gel
- Curlformers
- Optional: Ponytail hair bands to secure the roots
- Optional: Hooded dryer

Follow these steps:

1. Dampen hair with spray bottle containing water
2. Add holding product and/or oil
3. Add 8 or more small to medium size braids, twists or bantu knots
4. Add ponytail hair band to secure and lay down the roots
5. Allow hair to air dry or sit under a hooded dryer
6. Style as usual

Coach's Tip: This is a good "old school" way to do a blow out on damp to dry hair also. You do not have to use heat for this technique.

Stretch Hair with Bands

What you will need:

- Spray bottle containing water
- Oil and/or gel
- Moisturizer
- Hair bands
- Ponytail holders (medium and small)
- Boar bristle brush
- Scarf

Follow these steps:

1. Dampen hair with spray bottle containing water
2. Spray the edges making sure they are really damp
3. Moisturize the edges and exposed areas
4. Optional: Apply light oil or gel to the edges
5. Brush into a smooth ponytail at the back of the head
6. Add ponytail band
7. Brush the ponytail and add a band about ¼ inch from the first band
8. Add additional bands all the way down the ponytail to the end
9. Tuck your ends, twist it or leave it out
10. Smooth the edges
11. Wrap the hair with a scarf

12. Optional: Sit under a hooded dryer
13. Optional: Wear the hair banded or remove the bands

Coach's Tip: You can do 2 or more banded ponytails for a quicker drying process. You can also blow the hair out and/or style on this stretched out hair.

NOTES:

_____

_____

_____

_____

Stretch Curly, Q'coil, Twist Out or Braid Out Styles

What you will need:

- Bobby pins
- Thread
- Ponytail hair bands
- Flex rods or curlformers

Follow these steps:

1. Start on dry styled hair

2. Divide hair into 2 or 3 sections
3. Optional: Apply a light mist of leave-in conditioner or light holding spray
4. Start twisting from the back of the neck
5. Twist in a roll up towards the front of the head
6. Optional: Stop at the top
7. Optional: Twist to the end of hair and tuck into bantu knot or add ponytail
8. Secure with hair pins if needed
9. Apply scarf for 10 minutes or overnight

Coach's Tip: This works best on completely dry or 90% dry hair.

NOTES:

_____

_____

_____

_____

Stretch and Straighten Hair with Curlers

What you will need:

• Spray bottle containing water

- Oil and/or gel
- Curlformers
- Optional: Ponytail hair bands
- Optional: Hooded dryer

Follow these steps:

1. Dampen hair with spray bottle containing water
2. Add your holding product and/or oil
3. Add roller papers if needed
4. Add curlformers, rollers, perm rods or other curlers from the bottom of the hair up to the root
5. Allow hair to air dry or sit under a hooded dryer
6. Optional: Separate the hair to create volume
7. Style as usual

Coach's Tip: You can also use this method to twist small to medium sized sections of hair to the end before you do step 5, add your curlformers, rollers or perm rods to the ends. Also securing each sectioned piece of hair with a ponytail band can lay the roots down smoothly.

NOTES:

_____

_____

_____

How to create the deep wave bun

I get asked a lot about my bun. Anybody who knows me knows I have really thick dense hair. It's hard to imagine how I can actually lay it down. Well, I do have a few special things that I have to do in order to get that sleek, smooth look.

What you will need:

- Gel
- Spray bottle containing water
- Toothbrush
- Boar bristle brush
- Elastic hair bands
- Donut form

Follow these steps:

1. Start on damp washed or co-washed hair
2. Divide hair into 3 to 4 sections (back, middle, one in the top parted from ear to ear)
3. Start with the section in the back
4. Gel entire section, brush and band
5. Continue with the middle section
6. Gel entire section, brush and band it to the back section
7. Continue to the top section in the front
8. Optional: Divide the top into two sections to wear a part
9. Gel the front sections

10. Mold the hair back and ban it to the middle section
11. Wrap banded hair around donut evenly
12. Add a band around the donut
13. Smooth edges with a toothbrush
14. Wrap head for 20 minutes or overnight
15. Optional: Sit under cool dryer with head wrap for 25 minutes or until dry

Coach's Tip: The hair can also be divided into two sections, one in the front and one in the back or one on each side of the head. Do not pull elastic bands too tight; this will stretch out your natural wave pattern. Be sure to test out the gels based on how thin or thick your hair is. Refresh or re-do this once a week or as needed.

NOTES:

_____

_____

_____

_____

How to taper straight or wavy edges

Smoothing tapered edges will give any style a neat and manicured look.

Straight or Wavy Edges

What you will need:

- Ponytail band
- Gel
- Optional: Edge control
- Toothbrush
- Moisturizer cream
- Scarf

Follow these steps:

1. Apply gel or edge control product
2. Brush into the edges
3. Apply a small amount of super holding gel on top
4. Brush into hair
5. Shape edges
6. Wrap with a scarf to air dry
7. Optional: Blow dry

Coach's Tip: For fuller edges you can add dark spray semi-permanent hair color on your finger to dab on thin edges at the end of the process.

NOTES:

_____

_____

How to flat iron curly or straight hair

Natural or relaxed hair doesn't really need oil during the flat ironing process; it's optional. The hair will produce its own natural oil over time. *Always* deep condition or use a hot oil treatment prior to shampooing or after your shampoo or co-wash. If you follow this process, your straight style will last longer. For the best results, moisturize with a deep conditioner or light oils. Follow the detangle regimen in Chapter 4.

Flat ironing curly hair

What you will need:

- Ceramic flat iron
- Pressing product or serum
- Large paddle brush
- Soft boar bristle brush
- Rat tail comb
- Plastic cap
- Deep conditioner
- Optional: Oil

Follow these steps:

1. Start with the deep conditioner regimen and the blow out regimen prior to straightening
2. Take about 1/2 inch thick and 1 ½ inch wide sections of hair
3. Add a pressing product or serum to the parted strands (with a toothbrush, optional)
4. Glide the flat iron slowly down the strands from root to tip 1 to 3 times
5. Optional: Trim ends (see instructions for trimming natural or straight hair on page 49)
6. Use a paddle brush to wrap hair around the head
7. Use boar bristle brush to smooth the wrapped hair
8. Cover with clear plastic wrap and sit under hooded dryer 15 minutes
9. Optional: Cover with a wave cap to set overnight
10. Uncover hair and style

Coach's Tip: Setting the hair on magnetic rollers prior to flat ironing can lessen the amount of heat required during the process.

NOTES:

_____

_____

_____

_____

Hair growth tips

- Maintain a good healthy diet
- Master good hair care regimens and techniques
- Use protective styles during the harsh seasons
- Massage the scalp with oils
- Cover your hair while sleeping, swimming or working out
- Drink plenty of water

I really enjoyed putting this information together for you. I wrote the book that I wished was available when I was transitioning and struggling to maintain healthy hair. Now that you are armed with step-by-step guidance to care for your hair, recommend this book to your friends and family as the ultimate resource for helping them to care for their natural hair.

One thing I realized on this journey is that when the time comes for me to walk into paradise, I will only be able to take the hair that God has given me. I am so happy that I now know how to love and care for it.

Love Jehovah God first,
Your family next and
All of your neighbors
Don't forget to love YOU!

Want to contact me about the information in this book?
Email: contact@goodhaircoaching.com

The best compliment I can get is an amazing review, please be so kind as to leave a review on Amazon.

REFERENCES AND RESOURCES

Books

- *Better than Good Hair* by Nikki Walton
- *The Science of Black Hair* by Audrey Davis-Sivasothy
- *I Love My Hair* by Natasha Anastasia Tarpley and E.B. Lewis
- *Curly Girl Guide* by Lorraine Massey

Bloggers/Vloggers

- CurlBox.com
- Naptural85.com
- MahoganyCurls.com
- TarynGuy.com
- Curlynikki.com
- Heyfranhey.com
- NaturallyCurly.com
- BraidsbySheka.com

ABOUT THE AUTHOR

Meloney Washington is the founder of Good Hair Coaching. Meloney loves working with women, coaching other hair care professionals and giving lectures on natural hair care. This book was written for those women who are on the fence about how to transition or maintain their natural hair.

A former business and financial services professional, Meloney lives in Florida.

To connect with Good Hair Coaching, visit:

www.goodhaircoaching.com or
www.facebook.com/GoodHairCoaching